TRANSFORM YOUR BODY

12 Weeks to a New You

Martin Hutton

Contents

Chapter Seven: AND FINALLY………

- Sleep
- Hydration

RECIPES: (A few ideas to get you started…..)

- Simple scrambled eggs
- Tomato and chorizo salad
- Mackerel pate
- Broccoli cheese soup
- Carrot and sweet potato mash
- Cod with creamy leeks and bacon
- Chicken one tray bake

RECOMMENDED BOOKS:

- Some further reading

"I've always believed that if you put in the work, the results will come"

Michael Jordan

Introduction

WHAT IS A TRANSFORMATION?

This is the first question that I need to answer.

I have seen many gyms and trainers offer 12 week body transformations. They post the before picture at the start and then 12 weeks later they post a picture of the same person with a six pack.

If this is what you are after, then this book and my 12 week body transformation are not for you.

This person has dedicated 12 weeks to this. They have trained most days, sometimes twice a day, eaten exactly what they were told to eat, put this change before everything else and they have the results to show for it, which is excellent for them.

I do things differently. My 12 week transformation is intended to transform your body inside and out through developing your understanding of what you put into it and how to train effectively to enable you to transform how you feel and look.

This will enable you to make and see huge changes within 12 weeks but also give you the information to carry this on and maintain the changes you have made. *Maintenance* is the vital component.

For me, it is not just about working with people to change them for 12 weeks and then leaving them to it. I want you to still be eating, looking and feeling the same way in 5, 10, 30 years from now because you have grown to understand *why* you have made the changes that we will be implementing here.

It is about altering your attitude, your way of thinking and your knowledge as much as changing your body. Together we will change all of these things.

In this book, you will learn how to change your body shape by cutting fat and building lean muscle to give you a lean, athletic build.

I will also show you how you can have more energy and confidence whilst feeling the best you ever have and I will explain how you can do all this successfully while you are managing work and family commitments.

As I said, this book is not only about changing your shape. It is also about *maintaining* it for years to come.

The 12 week transformation is just the start and will give you tools to go on with your transformation for the rest of your life.

Chapter 1

MY
TRANSFORMATION
JOURNEY

Before I start, I want to make it clear that I am not a doctor nor a scientist. I am both a qualified personal trainer and ex chef and I combine my love of fitness and food in order to work with clients to help them transform their bodies inside and out.

I do not claim to know everything. I am constantly studying and learning and trying to improve my knowledge to push myself and my clients even further. However, I have the proof that it works. Firstly with myself, being the fittest, leanest, most energetic, successful and healthiest that I have ever been as I approach 40 and secondly my many clients who have implemented these changes and seen drastic transformations to their shape, fitness and health in only 12 weeks.

My Story

I have always been into sports and have kept fairly active over the years. However, like most people, working long hours and enjoying myself to excess took its toll and my fitness levels began to drop and I soon became unhappy with my shape.

I, like many people, went through the usual procedure of joining a gym, plodding on treadmills, lifting some weights, without proper guidance, eating more of what I thought (and was led to believe) were 'healthy foods' and reading fitness magazines to try and get ideas to follow. Basically I was doing all the things that I thought I was supposed to do to get results. I hated every minute of it and this was made all the worse for the fact that I was getting nowhere fast and my body was not changing.

All around me in the gym were people in the same situation. Every day I saw the same people, doing the same things and not looking particularly thrilled to be there.

Week after week, everyone was repeating this process and not getting the results they believed would come. Surely the whole essence of a gym is that it should be filled with fit, muscled, healthy people? All I could see were people in the same shape as me and none of us seemed to be changing.

My First Mistake

Having read the endless information available I thought I had the solution. Eat less and exercise more. This seemed to be the general consensus. Following this advice I cut back on fats and followed the low fat idea of eating as it seemed to make sense. So skimmed milk, more pasta, rice, bread, cereal and plenty of fruit were in along with diet juices.

A basic day would be cereal, orange juice and some brown toast for breakfast, pasta with a low fat sauce for lunch, chicken and rice for dinner, again with a low fat sauce, and snacks of fruits and low fat yoghurts. Surely this is the answer I thought. I will see some results now.

A few months later and still no difference. Even after a big change in the way I ate along with going to the gym 4 times a week, still nothing.

My next step was to take up running. I loved this, getting outside and enjoying the fresh air (probably the first sign that gyms just were not for me) and I did see a slight change in my body, not much, but change none the less and this gave me the incentive to continue. I entered into a 10k race and I enjoyed this so much that I was officially hooked.

Next I invested in a stationary bike that I could use at home. I used this daily, watching television as I cycled away, night after night. Again I saw some changes, lost some weight and was happy at the progress. I could feel my clothes getting slightly looser, my belt going down a notch. This is the way to do it I thought. I've cracked this, happy days!!

A Change Of Career

With a few changes in my life happening around this time, I fancied a career change. Based on my new found love for health and fitness, I looked into becoming a personal trainer. This way I could incorporate my new interest in running and exercise with my life long love of sport into my working life too.

At the beginning of the course we learned to measure body fat. No problem I thought, mine must be low, I have lost weight recently, let's do it. To my extreme shock my body fat was 24%, one of the highest in the group. How could this be? I was not fat, I had always been tall and thin, this couldn't be right. I believed that being skinny made me fit and healthy and being fat meant unfit and unhealthy. My lecturer explained I was what they call 'Skinny Fat'. Under lean but over fat, most of which was carried around the middle (he was spot on).

This panicked me as I thought I was healthy and thin and was doing everything right. I threw myself into the course, absorbing everything I could.

Upon gaining my personal training qualification, I began my new journey in earnest. 'The gym is your new home' I was told, get used to it. So I trained and began to see better results for myself and then started to pick up clients. Everything was good and I was moving in the right direction. However one thing was still annoying me and no matter how much I ignored this feeling, it was still there......... *I did not enjoy the gym.*

Now, you can understand my concern. I had just paid over three thousand pounds to become a personal trainer then realised I did not like gyms or even being in them.

This got me thinking that there must be another way to get fit, burn fat and build muscle. Something I can look forward to doing and which is enjoyable. I thought if I feel and think like this, I have to presume there are lots of people who feel the same.

Thinking back to previous times training in gyms, (I say training, but I now use that term loosely for what I had been doing), I remember the miserable faces of people just doing what they thought they had to, going through the motions of what they were told was the right thing and I realised I was not alone in my thinking that gyms just were not the place I wanted to be.

Thinking Differently

With my love of sports, I decided to research how the athletes I admired in sports such as tennis, boxing, basketball, American football etc, train day in, day out, in order to achieve the fitness and bodies they have. If I got bored training for an hour in these gyms 3-4 times a week, how did these people manage it 7 days a week for hours on end, month after month?? What was their secret?

I started spending many hours poring over books and the internet, soaking up information and techniques that athletes used. I found that they trained for a purpose, not just for show. Yes, I wanted the body, but I also admired other aspects of these people. Their athleticism, flexibility, endurance. I wanted all of this, not just to look good in a t-shirt, (though vanity was and still is high up my list for reasons to train and eat well!)

During my research I came across alternative methods such as battleropes, medicine balls, slam balls, TRX straps, sandbags and kettlebells. This type of training gives exactly what I was after, cutting body fat and building lean muscle while keeping me flexible and athletic. Where athletes had their reason to train (for their sport) I now had mine. To get fit for life and to be able to feel, look and operate at my best each and every day.

I started training this way and saw some results quickly. Although my weight did not go down (in fact I actually put on a few pounds) I could see my shape changing. My clothes sat differently on me. Instead of just hanging off me, I felt like I was now filling them and wearing them properly.

Again researching further into how these athletes trained, I noticed that a lot of their fitness sessions were quite short with the emphasis more on intensity. This was an eye opener as I had been programmed, like many of us, to think that an hour in the gym was the way to get in shape.

I then spent a lot of time researching this, poring over any studies and information that I could find relating to this and they all seemed to point towards high intensity interval training (HIIT) as the best way to burn fat and build lean muscle. This type of training went hand in hand with the new equipment and techniques I was using and so I switched to 30 minute sessions, with the emphasis on intensity. Before I started I was quite sceptical about this. How could I get fit in 30 minutes? It went against everything that I had learned and been taught, but putting this aside I pushed on with it.

Again, the results were immediate. The 30 minute sessions flew past but at the same time I felt that I had put more into and gotten more out of the session than any 60 minute plus session that I had ever done. My body fat was going down and my muscle mass was increasing. This felt strange, almost as though I was cheating. How could I be training less than ever but getting far better results ?

This prompted more investigation and I started to look at how trainers around about me trained. I noticed that they never used cardio machines. They never used the machines, yet encouraged gym members to do so. Gyms are 80-90% made up of cardio and weight machines, yet the fitness 'experts' never actually use this equipment for their own training. This got me wondering whether gyms were set up for clients to be successful. Is it any wonder I and many others spent years, not to mention money on membership fees, to spend time on treadmills and muscle isolating machines whilst getting nowhere yet were led to believe that if we kept going the results would come ?

This convinced me more that my type of high intensity training using kettlebells, ropes, sandbags and medicine balls was the way to go. Full body training was the best way to lose fat and build muscle. Using as many muscles as possible at once was the key whilst keeping the intensity up near maximum.

I have seen the results for myself. I am not just repeating what I have been told on a course or read in a book. I know it works as it has given me my best shape and fitness levels ever, even now in my late 30s.

These were the methods I started using with my clients. I trained them the same way I train myself. My client list became full with people like me. People who had become disillusioned with gyms, tired of the environment and of having to spend endless hours slogging away for little return. Clients started enjoying the sessions and the sensation of getting fit along with the feeling of more energy and the confidence that came with it. They were happy with the changes to their body shape.

Over time, my client list stayed full, retention was high and I actually had people waiting to train with me. Life was good.

Discovering The Importance Of Food

However, one thing bothered me and it was that although all my clients had told me they felt fitter than ever, had stopped worrying about losing weight and now worked on losing fat (which all had done), I still only had a few 'big transformations' from the people I worked with. I wanted all my clients to get stunning results, not just a few. I wanted all of them to have total transformations, slash body fat and build the body that they wanted.

Then I thought of myself again. I had travelled a long way on my fitness journey, but how much further could I take it? Yes, I was leaner than ever before, had more energy, was competing in races ranging from 10 km to 20 miles and getting top 10 finishes. But what now? What was my next step? What made the people finishing 8-9 minutes ahead of me able to do so? How could I take my transformation to that next level? What was I missing that I could adjust? This was when I seriously started to look at how I was fuelling my body and how my diet was affecting my results.

Again, I reverted to eating as the top athletes ate. If it was good enough for them it was good enough for me. Using myself as a tester for this, I'd give myself the proof that it worked and then use the same formula on my clients.

Although I was a 'healthy eater' as I thought, getting proteins and fats in my diet and keeping refined carbs to a minimum, I wanted more. I got as many books on the subject as possible and spent my time reading them cover to cover, fascinated at the amount of differing opinions on how to eat for optimal health.

So much contradictory information and alternatives made it clear why people get confused, overwhelmed and disillusioned. So many experts yet so many differing viewpoints. I had to find a way to simplify and correct this information for my clients.

The Truth Behind Low Fat Eating

One piece of information that stuck in my head was a report on obesity levels. (This is one bit of factual information that all experts agreed on.) In the 1970s obesity levels were under 3%, whereas now they were roughly 30% and rising. What had changed in this time? What was the big difference?? As I looked into this more I discovered that this coincided with when we had been encouraged to go low fat by 'health experts'.

In the late 70s/early 80s there was a big boom in the promotion of low fat eating. Fat was bad, it was reported and we were to stay away from it. Low fat yoghurts, ready made meals, low fat milks and creams were being pushed along with breads, pastas and rice until they became staples of our kitchen and formed the majority of our daily intake. Eggs were to be eaten minimally, nuts too as they were high in fat. Cut back on red meats, stay away from full fat milk and avoid butter. These were the foods that were doing the damage.

Avoid fat and avoid getting fat. This was the secret, so we were led to believe. Yet here we are 30+ years on and we are quickly becoming more obese and unhealthy than we have ever been.

This resonated with me and I began to look at my own diet and content more closely. I read numerous books on the effects of fat on the body and the now mounting research and evidence that suggested that low fat eating was not the way to go. They dispelled the innacuracies of the government food pyramid, explaining that it was badly designed and that the information and ideas given were highly inaccurate. Make the majority of your diet bread, cereals, pasta and rice they say. More of this than of fruit and vegetables? Keep meats, fish, eggs and nuts even smaller in proportion. They even taught this in schools and medical professionals encouraged patients to follow this route.

This is how we have been advised to eat, yet health and weight problems continue to rise. Something cannot be right.

My research continued and I began to look at how athletes eat to enable them to perform and train as they do at the highest level. I was amazed at what I found. We, myself included, were eating more 'energy foods' (carbohydrates) than top athletes. However these athletes then go on to train for their sport, working out in the gym and playing matches to burn this off, remaining active for 5/6 hours a day sometimes. Looking at my own eating, 'healthy' as it was and as fit as I was, I was still making mistakes and had room for improvement. Either that or I had to become a top sportsman and win major tournaments, so altering my eating was the more likely option!

Reading and discovering more about the effects of carbohydrates and sugar on the body was an eye opener. About how we had become so reliant on them after being told to cut back on our fat intake. How health problems have increased since these recommendations. How bread was higher in the glycaemic index (a ranking of carbohydrate in foods according to how they affect blood sugar levels) than chocolate bars and ice cream. How sugar causes many of the aches and pains we all take for granted (inflammation of the body).

Once again using myself as the tester, I set out to bring my sugar and carb intake right down, increase the fat content of my diet and keep the protein levels roughly as they were. I stuck to real foods - meat, fish, nuts, eggs, vegetables and fruit. I cut sugars and excess carbs (changed lentil soups for vegetable-based ones, added avocado to my breakfast and switched from semi or skimmed milk to full fat). Gradually I began to notice the changes and within 4 weeks the results were breathtaking.

Pains and stiffness that I had just put down to not stretching enough after training and getting older were gone. Every morning previously I would wake and take 10 minutes to loosen up, but not now.

Bloating and the discomfort in my stomach which I had long suffered from was a thing of the past. My stomach was now flatter than ever.

My energy levels went through the roof. Gone were my afternoon naps (which I had accepted as just being tired from early morning starts and late finishes and the energy I burned training). I slept better at night with no more broken sleeps, and I woke up fully charged for the day ahead.

As well as my energy levels being higher they were actually now more stable. The cravings that I had mid afternoon for sugar to keep me going had gone along with my need for a quick nap. I was actually now craving the olives, sundried tomatoes, nuts, carrots and guacamole that I had now become accustomed to snacking on. On top of this I had lost 4 pounds and I was more defined.

My one concern was the races that I took part in. I, like everyone else, had been taught to believe that we need all these carbs and sugar for energy, we cannot function properly without them and we certainly cannot exercise or run without them. The telling point would be competing in a major race a few weeks later. 20 miles and 200 obstacles. I had done it previously and found it very difficult - the most challenging thing I had ever done. Previously, I had 'carb loaded', filling up with cereal bars and pasta the morning of and night before the race. Now, on my new low sugar/carbs way of eating, basically losing all these 'energy foods', I took 50 minutes off my personal best. I felt lighter, leaner, fresher and more agile during the race and in general.

A few weeks later, after running my first marathon, I celebrated with a pizza. I had just run a marathon, so what harm could it do, I deserved it. However within twenty minutes of eating two slices of a '5 grain dough' pizza, I was doubled over in pain, my stomach was bloated and sore, I felt sluggish and sleepy and had what I can only describe as brain fog. Looking back, this was the first time I had eaten wheat in months and this was the effect. Had this been happening to me, to a lesser extent, on a daily basis before when I ate these foods? Because my body had been rid of it for so long and had become unaccustomed to having it, was this the real effect of this 'healthy eating' we have been advised to follow by government guidelines ?

Questioning What the 'Experts' Say

This is from the government website www.nhs.uk on their recommendations for healthy eating:

"Base meals on potatoes, bread, rice, pasta and other starchy carbohydrates. Choose wholegrain where possible.

Eat some beans, pulses, fish, eggs, meat and other protein. Aim for at least two portions of fish every week - 1 of which should be oily...

If you currently eat more than 90g (cooked weight) of red and processed meat a day...cut down to 70g."

So, we should base our meals on foods such as bread, pasta, rice and potatoes and not vegetables and fruits? Vegetables and fruits that are full of vitamins and minerals that our body needs in order to function efficiently and bread and pasta which contain, well, bleached flour and water. That's basically it.

We should eat *some* protein (something that is essential for building and rebuilding our organs, muscles, skin, hair, nails, bones and certain hormones). Cut down on red meat, 70g of it maximum, but feel free to eat more than that weight in pasta,bread and rice ?

I now understand why many people are confused by all the contradictory advice. That is the reason this book has been kept small. I have learned from speaking to my many clients over the years that all the information they hear on a daily basis can be overwhelming. So, for that reason, I have kept the book short and concise. I have included the evidence I found from my many months and years of reading and trial & error on myself in both my training and eating. I have failed many times and this has given me the keys to my success.

I have tried running, swimming and cycling. I have lifted heavy weights/ low reps and light weights/ high reps. I have tried every class from boxing to yoga and everything inbetween. I have tried high carb/low fat eating and tried high protein, high fat and no carb diets. I have tried protein shakes and supplements, having them in drinks, smoothies and soups. I have read numerous books from so called 'experts', medics and governmental advice. I have bought or tried every silly gimmick piece of equipment from ab crunchers to wobbly balls for standing on and even that scary machine that is meant to basically shake the fat from your body!

Keeping It Simple

However, my success came when I started using common sense and learning from the correct people. I started looking at the basic biology of our bodies, where we came from, what we are designed to do (be active using full body movements on a regular basis) and the foods our systems are designed to function on (natural foods not factory made creations).

It is all very simple. However, we are confused from the bombardment of information we receive on what we should do, how we should train, how long we should train for, what to eat and when to eat it. It is all too easy to be thrown by it all.

What we need to do is listen to the best source. Our body. Your body's opinion is the one that matters. It will tell you when it is hungry. It will tell you when it is full. It will tell you the foods it wants because if you put the wrong things in it, it will let you know with aches, pains and signs. It wants to move and if you do not move enough it will get stiff and sore.

It wants you to have energy, but if you do not have enough it is telling you you are not giving it the proper foods to achieve this. It will get leaner and it will build muscle if you do what it needs you to do. It will be tired if you do not sleep enough and it will give you signs when you don't hydrate it enough. Everything you need to know is right there. You have the information to hand. You just need to act on it.

I have kept this book intentionally short and free from jargon. As I said, we are overwhelmed by information on a daily basis and this is part of the problem. This book is clear and concise and gives you the tools to change your life in only 12 weeks.

So let's get into it!

Chapter 2

CHANGE OF LIFESTYLE

THIS IS NOT A DIET

This is not a diet, this is a change of lifestyle. This is a way for you to transform your body, inside and out in just 12 weeks. However, it is also designed to ensure you have the knowledge and power to *maintain* these changes for the rest of your life.

My goal is not to set you up to fail. I do not want my clients to have to stay with me for life in order to maintain their transformation. If they have to then I feel I have not done my job correctly. This is not some slimming club and you will not get certificates or awards. Your body will be proof of your success.

Losing weight is easy. Chances are if you are reading a book like this, you have lost weight before. Perhaps many times. However, like most people, you have probably put this weight back on, plus more.

With this 12 week transformation I will not only change your body but I will give you the knowledge and understanding of how training and eating combined correctly are the keys to both changing and then maintaining your reshaped body for the long term. You will understand *why* you should and should not eat certain foods to best fuel your body, not just blindly follow another fad way of thinking. You will understand *why* you need to train in a certain way at a certain intensity and not become dependent on someone telling you every week for the rest of your life.

It is important however that you understand this is a lifestyle change. It is not easy and will not happen overnight, but twelve weeks is a short amount of time to set yourself up for a successful and healthy future.

I want you to still be eating and training this way in 5, 10, 15, 20 years from now. I want you to maintain your new body shape and end all this yo-yo exercising and dieting. I want you to feel the benefits and never want to go back to your old shape and eating habits.

The best project you will ever work on is yourself. Investing in yourself will be the best time and money you will ever spend. Look at this as a changing of your ways. Go into it with an open mind and you will get the results your hard work deserves.

HOW MUCH DO YOU WANT IT?

Upon meeting with clients at the beginning of the process, to see if we are suitable to work together, I have to decide from speaking to them or by asking them straight out "How much do you want this?". I am only interested in working with people as dedicated to their 12 Week Transformation as I am. There is no point me working harder than any clients I work with.

I tell my potential clients about how they will need to:

- Train at intensity they are probably not used to. They need to get used to pushing themselves out of thier comfort zone.

- Commit to training twice every week minimum.

- Change their diets and try new foods and a new way of eating in general (for most).

- Commit to getting enough sleep, which may mean cutting back on time spent watching television or using social media.

- Cut out the sugars and refined carbs that are causing the problems for them.

At the end of this discussion I tell them that it will not be easy. Major changes never are. I explain that their goals are achievable, but only if they can decide how much they really want this. Is it worth the sacrifices?

You have to ask yourself the same questions.

Are you willing to cut back on drinking every weekend? Is it worth losing a few friends if you do not go out doing what they do as often?

What is more important, that extra five or ten minutes in bed each morning after hitting the snooze button or using that time to get up and make yourself a breakfast to kick start your day and set you up for success ?

Is that hour long television programme more important than cutting your body fat and regaining your confidence and self-esteem?

It is not easy to get the body you want. If it was, we would all have it. However, it is doable. Do you want to be like most people and just accept what you currently have as your lot or as your future? Or do you want to make the changes that could impact your life and transform you into the person you want to be?

These are the questions you need to ask yourself to decide if you are determined and focused enough to reach your goals. That day in the future will come. That day you have circled on your calendar, in twelve weeks time, will come. The day you are aiming towards, be it a birthday, Christmas, a holiday or a special occasion, it will come round. You have to decide if you are going to get to that day in the shape and condition you are in just now or if you are going to get to that day in the best shape of your life, feeling and looking great.

TAKE RESPONSIBILITY

Losing weight is easy. Keeping it off is the difficult part. That is why it is important that you understand this is a lifestyle change and not a 12 week 'diet to lose weight'. What this book does is explain to you why it is beneficial to eat and train this way so you understand what it does to your body. This means you can take responsibility for your body. It is helping you understand why:

- Exercising in short and intense periods is the way forward.

- Cutting back on nutritionally empty foods such as pasta, bread, cereals, rice and potatoes will slash your body fat level.

- Using weights to add muscle, and not sticking to long, slow cardio, will help burn fat.

- How you eat is more important than how much you train.

At the end of the 12 week transformation you should be fully equipped to understand *why* your body has changed and to carry on with the ways of eating and training that have taken you to these results.

The reason you will not slip back into your old ways is because instead of just being told to eat and not eat certain foods meaning your cravings stay with you, you will gain the knowledge as to *why* you should eat a certain way. If you understand that bread for example can cause inflammation within your body giving you the stiffness, aches and pains you may suffer and can cause bloating and fatigue, you will be less likely to go back to eating it as you did.

This is about learning and understanding the effects of training and eating to transform yourself inside and out and to carry this knowledge on into the years to come.

Take responsibility for your own body.

Chapter 3

THE KEYS TO YOUR 12 WEEK BODY TRANSFORMATION

WORK HARD and SMART

Only 20% of the results you want will be achieved in the gym.

80% of your success will be achieved outwith.

I am not a coach who goes for cliché motivational phrases, however the saying above is very relevant to any success you will get.

This is something that is *vital* to understand fully. *In the gym we are breaking our bodies, not building them.*

When we exercise, we break down muscle when we work at the correct intensity. This is why working out for 60-90 minutes is not the answer and why doing "just one more set" will not be beneficial. If we have worked at the proper intensity and have broken the muscles adequately then that is the job of the gym done. That is the 20%.

The 80%, where we build up muscle, happens in the hours and days after. If we eat correctly and rest adequately, then the muscles repair themselves stronger and bigger and we see the change in our body shape that we desire.

When clients say they want to lose weight, what they actually mean is they want to lose fat. Losing weight can mean a combination of fat, muscle and water coming off the body. So to ensure we are losing fat only, along with doing resistance training we need to eat sufficient amounts of protein, fats and quality carbs to help maintain and increase our muscle mass. This will give you the lean, athletic shape you want.

Protein also has the benefit of making us feel fuller for longer. Nutrient dense foods such as meat, fish, eggs, nuts, seeds etc keep us satiated longer and we are therefore less likely to be feeling constant hunger, which in turn keeps our blood sugar levels constant and therefore helps manage our cravings and in turn our shape.

Now let's say you currently train two to three times a week. In a perfect world that would be a good start. However, you eat AT LEAST four times a day. Breakfast, lunch, dinner and snacks, sometimes more. That is at least 28 times a week that you eat. So that is two or three sessions against 28 times eating each week. It's simple maths. More success (and also damage) can be achieved with the eating than the training.

Here is another example. Let's say you use a treadmill and run for an hour (or more) or burn about 400 calories. Sounds impressive. However when you look at this compared with food, 400 calories is basically one chocolate bar and one can of a sugary drink, which I could eat and drink within 5 minutes. So 5 minutes damage takes over an hour to work off (if we go by calories in against calories out to keep it simple just now). This shows the importance of food.

I tell my clients not to look at training as calories burned. At the end of a gruelling 30 minute training session when they are lying sweating, puffing and panting I explain that they have burned the equivalent of a mars bar. All that just to burn a bar of chocolate! Next time they go to eat a bar, they will think of that session and realise what it takes to reverse the damage of that sugar intake on their bodies never mind the damage it does to how they feel, their energy, their sleep quality etc.

Training has two functions:

1. It builds muscle.
2. It increases your cardiovascular levels.

However, while we will be building muscle, this will be hidden beneath the fat on our bodies. Until we burn this fat, predominantly through food, we will not see the benefits of these improvements. Yes, we will feel fitter, stronger and have more energy and stamina, but without the eating being correct, the transforming of our body just will not happen.

To reiterate, you break your body down in the gym and build it up elsewhere. If you understand this you will be ten steps ahead of the average gym goer.

Many gym goers have their training planned out ; what they will do on certain days, what areas of the body they are targeting and when. Some have it planned weeks, maybe months ahead. If you ask them what they are having for dinner that night, they have no idea. They concentrate 80% of their time and efforts on something that will affect 20% of their results and spend 20% of their time on the thing that will affect 80% of their success.

I spend 80% of my time on what I am eating. I plan ahead, cook in bulk then freeze meals and have snacks to hand so I am never caught out. I spend the majority of my time on what will give me the majority of the results I want and this is the secret.

So work hard and be smart and get the body you want.

THROW OUT YOUR SCALES

When people talk about losing weight, they don't really understand what this means. They say they want to lose weight, but this isn't what they actually mean.

What they want to lose is *body fat* not *body weight*. This makes using scales to measure progress useless (and very discouraging).

If you follow a calorie restricted diet then, yes, you more than likely will lose weight. If you join a slimming club then, again, it is more than likely you will lose some weight. However, if, for example, you lose 6 pounds then as much of it could be muscle as is fat.

We want to lose fat and maintain (or increase) muscle as it is vital we do this as we age, in order to maintain optimal health. We do this by using weights and resistance in our training (see my chapter on using weights for more information).

Have you ever seen someone who has lost a lot of 'weight' from going on some new fad diet?? Your first thought is that they look terribly thin, they have lost their shape, they seem to have excess skin, their face is drawn and they have aged. Well done to them for the effort involved in losing weight, but unfortunately a large chunk of this has been muscle. This is why they have lost that shape and seem to have skin hanging down as the muscle to hold their body in shape is no longer there.

This is why slimming clubs do not work. They promise that you will lose weight and technically they are not incorrect but, as we now know, we want to lose fat. You go along and lose 5-

6 pounds in week one (largely water). You are delighted so you follow the plan religiously, excited at what's to come. After week two, you lose 2 pounds. Okay, not bad, but a bit disappointing compared to week one. You were hoping for another 5-6 pound loss. However, you keep at it and after week three you lose......nothing. You are distraught. How did that happen? You followed the plan! Seven days of 'being good' and nothing to show. You are a bit disheartened so you have a bit of a cheat and have a takeaway or some cake to cheer yourself up. After week four you are a pound up! Demoralised, you walk away from it and that is you back to square one.

Telling people not to concern themselves with the scales is a daily occurrence for me and it is hard for people to break the habit, but doing so will help you reach your goals quicker and easier. Weight is a highly inaccurate way of tracking your progress and is the most likely way to jeopardise your hard work.

Two people could weigh 200 pounds and one could have 30% body fat and the other 10%. The scales cannot differentiate. Muscle is more dense than fat, so you could remain the same weight or lose less than you think you should, but see a massive change in your shape, in how clothes sit on you and how you look.

To track your progress take pictures at the start on day 1, front and side on, then again on day 28 and every four weeks thereafter. It's the same with clothes. Find something you don't wear often, see how it feels, how it sits on you, where it is tight and where it is loose then put it away for 28 days and try it on again. You will see and feel the difference and recognise the changes in your body in that time.

Another tip is to measure yourself, around the following areas, always at the fullest part:

- Chest, across the nipples
- Just under the pecs
- Waist, an inch above your belly button
- Hips at the widest part
- Thighs at the thickest part
- Calves at the thickest part.

Measuring your progress is one of the most important parts of your transformation. Do it correctly and you are well on the way to achieving your targets.

SET TARGETS

What exactly do you want to achieve? The very first thing you need to do is decide this.

Do not be vague. Do not just say to lose weight/fat and get fitter etc. We need to be more definitive in our answer. For example, 'I want to drop a dress size within 10 weeks'. The more definitive, the more chance that you will reach your goal.

What I use with clients is SMART goal setting and this will help you change your goals from "I want to lose some weight and get thinner" to "I want to transform my body by burning one and a half stone of fat and building 6-8 pounds of lean muscle in the next 12 weeks before I go on holiday".

This will make your targets more structured and trackable and having a deadline really focuses the mind.

Your goals must be:

Specific: What exactly do you want to achieve?

Measureable: How are you going to track this? My clients use weekly food diaries, take pictures every four weeks to monitor change in body shape and use certain clothes to again measure, on a four weekly basis, changes in shape.

Attainable: Set goals that are realistic, otherwise you only end up despondent and this is what leads to failure. Make your goals challenging but achievable and you are more likely to be successful.

Reachable: How are you going to reach your goals?

With my clients we agree that they will try cooking and eating more fresh, natural foods, that they will try a new food at least once a week, that I will provide them with recipes to try, that they will train twice a week, that they will drink more water and that they will cut back on sugars. Again having these goals and being accountable makes the process easier and gives more chance of success.

Timed: When are we reaching these goals by??

This is why saying "I want to lose some weight" is a sure way of failing. It is too vague. To have no deadline makes it easier to give up, to have a day where you do not feel like training or eating properly and to think a day off won't do any harm.

When you have a set date by which you need to complete your target, i.e. a holiday, wedding or Christmas party, then you are more likely to stick to your plan as that date gets ever nearer.

DO NOT COUNT CALORIES

One of the other great myths of cutting body fat is that all calories are equal, which encourages people to restrict calories thinking it will get them the results they want.

Some facts:

Carbohydrates have 4 calories per gram
Protein has 4 calories per gram
Fat has 9 calories per gram

Simple maths would have us believe that eating less fat (9 calories per gram) and more carbs (only 4 calories per gram) will have us lose weight and give us the body shape we want, right?

So we eat low fat cereal, low fat yoghurt, skimmed milk, low fat ready meals, bread/pasta/rice/potatoes (all low fat foods). These foods make up the majority of our daily/weekly food intake and yet obesity levels are at their highest levels ever (and rising).

A large portion of our body is made up of fat (our brain is 60% fat). We have such things as essential fats and proteins, these are fats and proteins that we MUST GET FROM OUR FOOD because the body requires them for good health and can not synthesise them. There are however NO ESSENTIAL CARBOHYDRATES (though this is not to say do not eat carbs, we will come to that later). Yet we are being pushed to follow a low fat (and in turn high carbs and sugar) way of eating.

Going by this logic, eating a chocolate bar (roughly 260 calories) would be better than eating an avocado (up to 300 calories, the majority of them from fat) as it has less calories.

A prime example of how calorie counting is ineffective would be looking at athletes. Many of them consume 10,000 to 12,000 calories per day yet are not overweight. Yes they are training and competing on a daily basis and need extra calories going in to counter the energy they are using. However if you consider that running a marathon for an average person will burn around 3,500 calories, this means they would have to be doing the equivalent of three to four marathons each day to burn this off, which of course no one does.

What we need to look at is the quality of the calories we put in our bodies.

QUALITY MORE THAN QUANTITY

The quality of what you eat is more important that the quantity of what you eat.

2,000 calories gained from bread, pasta, cereals, rice, biscuits etc will have a totally different influence on your body shape and how you feel than 2,000 calories gained from fresh fish, meats, vegetables, avocados, nuts and fruits for example. So hopefully this helps dispel the calorie counting notion.

The quality of what you eat is the key to fat loss (and maintaining this long term). Your body needs certain vitamins and minerals from foods to enable it to function properly.

When we eat bread, pasta, cereals, cheap chocolate and sugary drinks our body (to keep it simple) says "Okay, you have given me something, but it doesn't contain what I need, so give me more, until I get what I need". This is why we are hungry shortly after eating these 'empty foods' and then we crave more and end up eating more of the same foods (as they are most convenient) and the whole process begins again as our body is never being given what it wants, but is constantly being given 'something'.

When we eat ' nutrient dense foods' such as meat, fish, nuts, fruit and vegetables, our bodies receive everything they need. They are satisfied so they do not go looking for more until they need it, until they have processed and suitably disposed of what they have been given. This keeps you full for longer and therefore reduces the urge to snack and binge.

A good indicator of how good certain foods are for you will be how much the supermarkets charge for them. Avocados are the new super food and the price has rocketed. Quinoa is deemed the same, now so much more expensive than a few years ago. Steak, salmon, sea bass, free range eggs, quality nut butters, coconut oil, olive oil, raspberries, strawberries and blackberries, for example, are all what you would call fairly expensive in relation.

Compare that with how cheap pasta and rice are. Cheap chocolate compared with real cacao, crisps compared to nuts, potatoes compared to tomatoes and peppers.

If these foods were so good for us do you not think the supermarkets would be charging top price for them?

The key is to listen to your body and give it what it wants.

VALUE YOUR BODY AND HEALTH

Following on from the previous section about the quality of foods, the main response I receive when I tell people that pasta, rice, potatoes, bread etc should be replaced by fresh meats, fish, fruit and vegetables is "It's expensive to buy that kind of food...".

This is somewhat true, quality in anything is not cheap. However, this is to give you ultimate health and wellbeing, so surely the added cost is well worth it?

When we have an issue with our cars, we go to the garage. After a check up we are told it will cost 'x' amount to repair it and bring it up to standard. So we pay and off we go with our car. However when it comes to our health and what we put inside our bodies, we hesitate at having to pay 'x' amount to repair and bring our bodies up to standard. Our cars take precedence over our bodies.

We do the same with furniture. We go and replace our two year old settee and spend thousands on a new one without giving it a second thought. Our beds however, we have had for 10 years and cost roughly £200-500. The place where we sleep, recover and repair our bodies is not considered at the same level of priority as the thing we sit on for a while to watch television.

We do not flinch at paying £20 for a takeaway meal for two on a regular basis, but grumble at buying fresh foods that maybe cost a pound or two more than the frozen or processed varieties. For that £20 we could buy quality, natural foods that would do us four or five quality meals.

To fully transform our bodies we need to re-evaluate our priorities. We need to invest in ourselves, put ourselves first and understand that we only get one body and we need to maintain it to the best of our abilities in order to get longevity and enjoyment from it.

Can you really put a price on getting the maximum enjoyment from your life and extending it as long as possible ?

ENJOY FOOD!

So far we have spoken about the effects food has on our body shape and well - being and this is important. However, sometimes we overcomplicate things.

Eating is something we will do 3 or 4 times a day, every day. It should be fun. It is to be enjoyed and celebrated. Eating is a pleasure and should be something we look forward to.

If we learn to enjoy food and not just see it as an inconvenience that 'we need to do' to function it becomes easier. Think European, where eating food is seen as a major part of the day, something to be enjoyed with family and friends.

People think of healthy eating as dull, boring and a chore. What is more enjoyable for breakfast, buttery scrambled eggs with some chives or a bowl of cornflakes? Dinners of dried pasta (with a use by date of 3 years away) with a shop-bought sauce or leeks and bacon cooked with cream and topped with fresh, well-seasoned fish?

Don't use time as an excuse (the two meals above can be made in 5 minutes). Make time, invest time in your body, include your family and let your children eat this way so they learn these habits, and you will get the overall reward back tenfold.

It is all a big circle. Eat better and you will feel better. If you feel better, you will have more energy and you will be able to train harder, giving you better results. Better results give you more encouragement to keep going as you see and feel the benefits.

Eat better, train better, sleep better, look better, feel better and so on. It is all about getting into good habits and then it will become a way of life for you and you will not want to go back to where you came from.

PREPARE FOOD IN ADVANCE

A big key to succeeding in your fat loss goals is preparing meals in advance. As I said earlier, what you eat is where you will see 80% of your success, so having your meals planned and prepared is essential.

As touched on previously, I see gym goers training 4, 5, 6 times per week for 60+ minutes. When I speak to them they have their routine planned, they know what they are doing today, the next session, sometimes they have it all planned out even weeks ahead. When I ask what they are having for dinner in about two hours time they have no idea. What did you have for breakfast? I just grabbed a cereal bar because I was in a hurry/I was running late/I cannot get myself up out of bed in the morning to make anything as I like an extra 10 minute snooze are the most common replies.

This will to lead to failure, no argument. Understanding that 80% of change comes from what you eat is essential to your success. I cannot emphasise this enough. We spend endless hours of hard work on the part that is contributing 20% to our success - the training. We travel to the gym, get changed, train, have a shower, travel home - all very time consuming. We do this 3, 4, 5 times a week. Yet the part that will contribute to

80% of our success we barely spend any time worrying about at all.

Personally, I spend 4-5 hours each Sunday on my day off preparing my food for the week between shopping, cooking and freezing my meals. I am busy and do not have the time to spend each day making breakfast, lunch, dinner, snacks etc 7 days per week. I dedicate a good part of Sunday to preparing for the week ahead, keeping any need for cooking during the week to a minimum.

Firstly I create a plan of meals for the week ; where I will be on what days and what I will need for each day. Then when I know my menu, I write a shopping list of everything I need to be able to make those dishes. Next, I spend a few hours preparing. Basically running it like a restaurant, prepping as much as I can in advance, so that it is only a matter of reheating or finishing it off come the time I am ready to eat. Once my meals are prepared and cooled, I portion them up and freeze for later in the week and keep some in the fridge for the next couple of days.

While my food is cooking, I am preparing my other ingredients for the week, chopping my vegetables and grating cheese and making dips and dressings to use with my meals and snacks during the week.

Preparation is the key.

Chapter 4

UNDERSTANDING FOOD

THE MYTH OF LOW FAT FOOD

Eating fat does not make you fat.

Eating low fat foods to lose fat is possibly the biggest myth in the fitness and fat loss industry.

As a chef I was told that flavour comes from three things : fat, salt and sugar.

Foods that have had fats taken out are bland as the flavour in the food is in the fat. Therefore shops would be selling you bland products and you would not buy them. So to replace this missing flavour they fill them with sugars, to sweeten them up.

This is the reason you will find sugars in ketchup, soups, ready meal lasagnes, yoghurts and biscuits. All correctly advertised as low fat, but the sugar content is frighteningly high and excess sugars in the body eventually will become fat.

Quite simply if you have neither fats nor sugars you have no real flavour.

The boom on low fat foods has been ongoing since the early 80s (when obesity was around 3%). In that time it has risen to around 30%, which can surely be no coincidence.
This became the launch pad for the low fat food craze that took people from eating nutrient dense foods such as eggs, meats, nuts etc and had them eating more processed, high sugar foods, such as low fat yoghurts, pasta and bread.

These reports denigrated certain foods such as eggs, one of the most beneficial foods you can eat, and blamed them for many ailments such as high cholesterol. Although research has now shown this not to be the case, eggs became the demon of the food world and we were told to eat these sparingly without any proof as to why, even though they have been shown to have huge nutritional value.

Manufacturers started removing fat from their products to go along with these guidelines then discovered that there was no flavour to their foods without it. It tasted bland. So what was the next best thing and cheap to keep the cost down? Sugar to sweeten it up.

So, if you see 'foods' with low fat stamped on them you will find them mostly filled with sugars i.e. low fat yoghurts. Seen as a healthy option they can contain up to 20 grams of sugar which is the equivalent of more than half a can of a sugary drink.

It is important that you question everything. Do not just take it for granted when you read or hear something. Don't believe low fat is bad? If we go on the assumption that you are looking to lose fat (i.e. you are reading this book) then complete a food diary for a week and go over it. Is it full of red meats, eggs, nuts, avocados, oily fish and seeds (all 'high fat' foods)? Or is it full of low/no fat foods such as pasta, bread, rice, potatoes, yoghurts, skimmed milk, cereals, crisps and biscuits?? Do not take it from me or from any other reports as to what is fact. Just look at your own body.

WHY FAD DIETS DO NOT WORK

As said before, losing weight is easy to do, we have all done it, but maintaining it is the hard part.
Do these fad diets work? Yes they will lose you *weight* and that is what they promise, so technically they are not lying. However, if you want to keep that weight off, that is another question.

Time and time again I see fitness centres, trainers and slimming clubs who post before and after pictures of clients who lose weight and that is great, the person is happy with their new body, job done. However, what we never see is how that same person looks a further three months on. Or a year later. Or five years later. Are they still the same size and shape? Have their health and fitness improved? Did they receive the information to continue their transformation journey successfully into the future?

I have a diet, but I am not on a diet. We all have a 'diet'. The *first* dictionary definition of a diet is :

The kinds of food that a person, animal, or community habitually eats.

My way of eating has gotten me to a certain body shape and fitness level that I am more than happy with, but I have never went without anything and never craved anything. That is where the success lies, the long term success that few of these 'diets' (*second* dictionary definition : A special course of food to which a person restricts themselves, either to lose weight or for medical reasons) provide.

Regarding food, some of the first things I ask any new client are ; What are your non-negotiables? What are the foods that you cannot do without? What are the foods that you really love? For me, they are chocolate and ice cream. Now as I said, I am more than happy with my body shape, fitness and health. I am the best I have ever been. Could I be even better? Yes, of course. If I cut out chocolate and ice cream, say for three months. My fat levels would drop even further, I'd be leaner, my muscle tone would be even more defined and I would be taking in less sugar, which as we now know would be a good thing for my body.

Great. The 'diet' (second dictionary definition) worked.

And if I stay off these two things, my body shape will remain the new way it is, however the chances of me staying off these two things after three months are non-existent (actually the chances of me staying off them for the initial three months are non-existent!). This means my body will revert back to the shape it was before I did all this, yo-yoing up and down.

So I never gave these items up. I ate them in moderation and controlled my portion sizes. And this is what you must do also.

Firstly, name your non-negotiables. Let's say, like me, that one of these is chocolate. Chocolate is an empty carb, supplying my body with false energy and little else, the same as pasta, bread, potatoes and sugary drinks. I need to decide what I want more, these items or chocolate. It's a no brainer for me, so I don't eat them. Next, chocolate or rice? Or cereal? Cereal bars?

Noodles? No brainer. You get the idea. It is about deciding what you want, what you cannot do without and keeping that and getting rid of the other items that are doing the damage.

It is always an eye opener for a client when I explain the items doing the damage then ask "Do you love eating that?" "Not really" is the usual reply. So why are you eating it daily then? Do you love cornflakes? No. Cereal bars? No. Low fat yoghurts? No. How about crackers that you eat every tea break? Or the rice, pasta and potatoes you have every day, do you love eating those? No, not really.

What we do first is get rid of the items that we do no care about and see the difference that makes to our shape and energy levels while keeping the items we love to eat, the things we derive real pleasure from and making sure we keep them but in controlled portions.

SUGAR

Also known as sucrose, corn sweeteners, high fructose corn syrup, dextrose, glucose, lactose and maltose to name but a few. A huge cause of the health problems we face today.

Over the past couple of hundred years, the amount of sugar that we have added to our diet is frightening and this has coincided with the rise in many illnesses and health issues that are prevalent today.

This is not only from the simple sources we all know about such as chocolate bars and sugary drinks. Bread, potatoes, rice and crisps are starchy foods that the body breaks down into simple sugars and they can make our blood sugar surge and crash like pure sugar can. Highly refined starches like white bread, crackers, white rice and pasta are the worst.

Sugar is everywhere and in everything that we eat, in many foods that you would never dream it was in. It has been covered up by the whole 'Fat makes you fat' myth that has been encouraged for the past 40 years and this has taken away the attention from the real culprit of our many ailments, *sugar.*

It is surely no coincidence that our ancestors' sugar intake was minimal and many of the illnesses we now see on a regular basis were not around back then. Sugar was found in fruit and honey along with vegetables, but the effects were minimised by the water, fibre, vitamin and nutrient content of these foods. We are eating less and less of these foods now and more of the foods above that have little to none of these added extras in them.

The key to your weight loss is here, in curbing your sugar intake and realising the damage being done to our bodies by our overindulgence in it.

We will go into this in more detail in the next few chapters.

BREAKING THE SUGAR CYCLE

Put into simple terms, carbohydrates are sugars and starches and these are absorbed quickly which is the reason why we get that almost instant energy surge when we eat foods such as chocolate, cereals, breads etc. Basically they are energy foods and do nothing more for the body than give us energy in one form or another.

When our sugar levels go up from these foods a hormone called insulin is released which then goes to work to quickly lower the levels of sugar in our blood to a safe, normal level. When this happens and the levels of sugar go down rapidly we feel weak and tired and we grab for a quick, sugary snack to boost our energy levels back up and so the whole cycle starts again.

Put simply:

Our bodies cannot cope with the amounts of sugar that we are putting into them.

The excess sugars are then stored as fat, predominantly around the waist and hips, which is a problem area for many and this is the reason why.

The answer is to keep our insulin levels at an even level throughout the day and the way to do that is to cut back on the refined carbohydrates and sugars from foods such as breakfast cereals, bread, pasta, ready meals, sugary drinks, cheap chocolate, pastries etc. Now this is not to say that we should stop the intake of carbohydrates. NOT ALL CARBOHYDRATES ARE THE SAME. They are not the enemy as all fruit and vegetables are carbs. It's making sure we are choosing the correct carbs.

The energy provided from a bowl of berries is very different from the energy we get from the foods mentioned previously.

We hugely overestimate the amount of these 'energy foods' we need. We mistake being busy with being active. Yes, we are all rushing about dealing with work, kids and everything that comes with it, but mostly we are doing these things without exerting much energy. We drive to work/get the train or bus, we have (most of us) jobs at desks or jobs which do not include tremendous amounts of physical exertion all day, we sit and eat dinner, then maybe we relax in the evening and watch television before bed. A busy day, yes, but not particularly physically exerting.

An eye opener for me was on researching the diets of sportsmen and women that I admired and finding that my diet was higher in 'energy foods' than these people who train 5-6 hours a day and compete regularly in their chosen fields. I was eating more energy foods than someone winning Wimbledon! As stated, carbohydrates are needed to some degree, so it is not about cutting them out altogether, it is about getting the balance right and understanding good carbs from bad carbs.

HIDDEN SUGARS

One of the reasons people struggle to get significant results when eating 'healthily' is that we are misinformed to what can actually be classed as healthy foods.

On a weekly basis I have new clients start and we complete food diaries to get a starting point for their transformation. It is normally followed by the sentence "My eating is quite good, it's the exercise that is the problem with me". However, even with this 'healthy eating' they are not seeing the results they want, leading to them becoming demoralised and going back to their old habits because "What's the point?"

We all know what unhealthy foods are. When I ask clients, the standard responses are pizza, biscuits/cakes, crisps, alcohol, takeaways, chocolate and ice cream. All valid foods to be aware of and keep to a minimum and most people do this when trying to cut fat.

When people cut out these items they see changes to their body but eventually these changes will level out and they will remain the same. This is where the frustration kicks in as to why they are not getting results when they are "being good".

The answer is in the *hidden sugars* that we are consuming every day, blindly, without even knowing, in foods such as yogurts, breakfast juices, cereals, ready-made sauces, ready meals etc. As well as these there are foods that have the same effect on your body as sugars do such as pasta, bread, rice and potatoes.

These are the foods that are doing the damage to us.

So when we are eating 'healthily' our day's eating may be roughly as follows:

- A breakfast consisting of cereal (high sugar), skimmed milk (removed fat, replaced with sugar) and dried fruit (intense sugar as water has been removed) with a flavoured yoghurt (high sugar).

- A lunch of pasta (bleached flour and water) with a shop-bought tomato sauce (surprisingly high sugar content for a vegetable-based sauce).

- A dinner made up of rice (starch = sugar effect), chicken (good protein) and some vegetables (nutrient-dense carbs).

- Snack of fruits (an excellent source of vitamins and minerals, but also high in sugar depending on fruits eaten and amount).

On paper this looks good, but it is totally imbalanced; there is an excess of sugar with only a couple of decent protein sources all day and very little of the necessary fats our body needs.

These foods that we are told are healthy and make up the bulk of our diet are doing us serious damage. The glycaemic index (GI) is a rating system for foods (from 0 to 100) containing carbohydrates. It shows how quickly each food affects your blood sugar (glucose) level when that food is eaten on its own. As we know from the previous chapter, keeping our blood sugar levels consistent is the key.

However, when you look at the GI you will find the following items rate alarmingly high:

Potatoes (85), cornflakes (77), white bread (69), rice (87), crackers (74), brown bread (67)

At the same time, cola has a rating of 63 and a chocolate bar is 49.

So you can see that our 'healthy eating' is really what is doing the damage, with potatoes and cereals having more of a negative effect on us than fizzy drinks and chocolate!

What we need to work on is getting a balance of real foods into our diets. Real foods that give our bodies the vitamins and minerals they need to function properly.

EMPTY FOODS IN MORE WAYS THAN ONE

Have you ever eaten a piece of cooked pasta on its own? Or a spoonful of rice? Or a dry slice of bread? Most people have not. There is a reason for this. These foods are bland and tasteless. Yet they make up the majority of our diet on a daily basis. This is the most frustrating part of my job and as a food lover. *We are actually getting fat by eating foods that we do not even like.*

When people say they love pasta and couldn't do without it, I ask if they have ever eaten plain pasta. Of course not. Why? Because it has no flavour, why would you? It is white flour and water mixed together with part of an egg to bind it. That's it. If that was mixed in a glass and you were offered it to drink you would understandably refuse. Same with bread. We spread butter, meat, salad, cheese, mustard, anything on it really. Most bread has little taste to it. It is there purely to hold the filling, where the flavour and taste is. Pasta is just the carrier for the sauce, which is where the flavour is, where the enjoyment comes from.

Potatoes, we put butter and herbs on, or we make a filling like tuna mayonnaise to put on top of a baked potato. When we have curry, we mix in the rice with the chicken and sauce. Or we get fried rice (they need to fry it in oil to give it some flavour).

These foods are just for bulk, added to make the meal go further. They bring nothing to the dish bar bulk. Experiment with your food, try different things and keep the variety.

Try baked sweet potato or try a bowl of broccoli with a sauce and parmesan cheese on top instead of pasta.

Change your thinking, make yourself try something new every week and extend your repertoire of meals. Variety is important. It will prevent you from getting bored and going back to your old way of eating.

ALWAYS QUESTION INFORMATION

Question everything.

Clients come to me, they train and take on board what I am saying and this is great, easy for me. At the same time, in conversations with a lot of clients I hear of exercises they have been told to try at a fitness class or by someone in the fitness industry. Or I hear of a new diet or super food that we are being told to eat and I am asked my opinion on it. And what I always say to my clients is this ; question the person telling you this. Make them work for your trust.

This includes me. I tell my clients to question everything I say ; to push me, ask me why we are doing a certain exercise, make me tell them why it is beneficial and what gains they are going to see from it. When I suggest my way of eating and what foods to eat and to avoid, push me as to why. Why is this good for me ? Why will that not do my body any good ? Is this way of eating balanced and will it give me everything my body needs ?

This is how you find out the people you should and should not be listening to. If they cannot tell you what benefits you will gain from a certain exercise then maybe they are not the person to be listening to. If they cannot tell you why you should eat this and not that then maybe this is not the person you should be taking food advice from.

I see people advocating diets and ask them "Will that give me all the vitamins and nutrients I need? Is there enough protein for me to maintain and build muscle? Are there enough fats in this to give my body what it needs?"

Same with exercise. Always be challenging "What is the benefit of this move ? What area am I working? What exactly is this doing for me?"

I have seen people jog on a treadmill as a warm up to lifting weights. How is this preparing your muscles to lift weights? Would a runner lift some weights as a warm up to run a race? No. They would mimic similar moves they are going to make in their main activity at a more gentle pace. This is the whole essence of a warm up.

Why would a nutritionist suggest eating pasta is healthy? Pasta is mostly white flour mixed with some water and part of an egg to bind it as we now know, so where are the health benefits from that? What exactly does our body get from this?

Always question what you are told before doing it. Make sure you are getting value for your money and value for the time you are investing.

Chapter 5

UNDERSTANDING WHAT YOUR BODY NEEDS

WHY WE NEED TO EAT FAT

Fat is not something to avoid or be scared of. In fact it is necessary to our wellbeing.

IT IS ESSENTIAL for:

- Growth and development,
- Providing energy,
- Protecting our organs,
- Maintaining cell membranes,
- Helping the body absorb and process nutrients, and
- Helping the body burn fat.

Fat also keeps you feeling fuller for longer, preventing those urges to go and grab some quick (convenient) snack, which is rarely the healthy option.

The vitamins A, D, E, and K are all fat-soluble, meaning that the body can't absorb them without fat. Therefore if your body isn't absorbing these nutrients properly, vitamin deficiencies will result which can cause dry skin, bone issues and muscle pains.

WHY WE NEED PROTEINS

Proteins are part of every cell, tissue and organ in our bodies. It is essential that we get enough of them from our diets for our bodies to function properly. They consist of chains of amino acids which are the building blocks of muscles, blood, skin, hair, nails and internal organs.

Too low an intake of protein can cause issues with your hair, nails and skin and lower your immune system making you more susceptible to picking up illnesses. It will result in muscle loss. Your body doesn't store protein the same way it stores energy in fat cells, so daily protein intake is necessary.

So we can see from the two previous sections that protein and fat have many essential functions within the body. We MUST get these two macronutrients in order to function properly. Now let us look at carbs...

WHY WE *DO NOT* NEED EMPTY CARBOHYDRATES

Our bodies can only hold a certain amount of carbs, thought to be between 1600 and 2000 calories worth. Most of us, even the most lean amongst us, store upwards of 40,000 calories worth of fat.

Put simply we have a limit to the amount of calories our body can take and use efficiently. This is where the big mistake is. We are totally unbalanced in our food intake.

Put very simply any carb intake after the 2000 or so calorie limit has to either be burned or it turns to excess fat. The macronutrient that we are least equipped to carry is the one that we eat the most of. The macronutrient that our body is best designed to carry is fat and this is the thing we have been advised to eat less of.

This is why we must limit our intake of sugars and refined carbs as there is nowhere for them to go. Either that or you need to start running a marathon each day to come close to burning off what you are taking in!!

Carbs are nothing more than energy. That's all they provide your body with, nothing more, unlike fats and proteins as discussed above.

As said before but worth repeating, it is all about giving your body what it needs, so let's talk a bit more about this and take it further to demonstrate exactly what we need to feed our body for optimum efficiency.

WHAT YOUR BODY WANTS AND NEEDS

So far I have kept this book quite simple as I believe much of the information around on the subject of fitness and fat loss is unnecessarily overcomplicated.

However, I think it is essential to go into a bit more detail to fully understand and get the most success out of your transformation that you can. This was what helped me take my understanding to the next level and with it my fitness and body shape, so here goes.

So far we have stuck to discussing the macronutrients; fat protein and carbs. However, to fully understand them, we need to break them down even further into micronutrients to understand the difference between *'good'* carbs, proteins and fats and *'bad'* carbs, proteins and fats.

Your body is an amazing thing. It takes all the food that you put into it, breaks it all down and reconstructs it as cells and energy that you need to function on a daily basis. However your body can only work with what you give it and this is why it is essential that you give it what it wants and needs. What it needs are micronutrients. These are what enable your body to function and you to have the shape, fitness and health that you want. It gets these micronutrients from breaking down the macronutrients you feed it. These micronutrients include potassium (bananas), zinc (beef), calcium (spinach and milk), vitamins B (eggs) & C (peppers, oranges and broccoli) and iron (nuts, seeds, seafood and dark chocolate!) to name but a few.

Foods high in calories (macronutrients) but low in vitamins and minerals (micronutrients) are what we would call 'empty' foods. These are what confuse your body. It understands that it has been given something to process. However it is not what it needs and therefore it craves the necessary foods full of what it does need, sending you hunger signals, causing you to eat more (usually more of the wrong foods) and so the cycle continues. Foods that are full of these necessary vitamins and minerals are what are known as 'nutritionally dense'.

Your intake of these essential micronutrients varies greatly depending on the quality and quantity of food that you eat. Fish, pasta and a banana are not just food to fill you up. They are broken down by your body and then redistributed and used for what it needs. If the foods you give it do not contain the necessary micronutrients then that is when the trouble starts.

Processed foods on the whole are higher than natural foods in macronutrients and lower in micronutrients. This is because in the processing of food to give it a longer shelf life and to produce it on bulk to keep it cheap, many of the nutrients and minerals are stripped from it. Freshly made bread is like a rock the next morning yet bread we purchase from supermarkets is still soft up to a week later. What is being done to our foods to make them this way? If food can sit in your cupboard or on a supermarket shelf for a year or more without deteriorating, why would we think that our bodies can break it down and use it for good?

This is why we must avoid, as much as possible, cereals, breads, pasta, rice, sugary drinks and snacks and try to make the majority of our diet up from fruit, vegetables, fresh fish, meats and eggs along with nuts and seeds to get the results we desire.

WHAT SHOULD YOU EAT?

VEGETABLES: Vegetables should form the basis of everyone's diet as they are dense in nutrients and vitamins. The usual response that I hear here is "But I don't like vegetables....".

There is such a vast array of vegetables that there must be some you will find that you can/will eat. We are guilty of thinking that vegetables and salad end with some lettuce and tomatoes. Vegetables are available in such abundance and they vary so much in flavour that you will find some to suit your tastes.

Another bonus is that they can be consumed in vast quantities compared to 'empty' carbs. For example 100g of pasta contains more than five times the amount of carbs that the exact same weight of broccoli does and bread has more than four times the amount of grams of carbs than an identical measure of carrots (source:*www.caloriecount.com)*

Therefore we can see that it is quality not quantity that matters as the same portion size of different foods can vary greatly in what they provide for your body.

Examples of vegetables to try include;

Celery, tomatoes, bell peppers, onions, leeks, green onions, eggplant, cauliflower, broccoli, asparagus, cucumber, cabbage, sprouts, artichokes, lettuce, spinach, collard greens, kale, beet top, mustard greens, swiss chard, watercress, turnip greens, seaweed, endive, rocket, bok choy, carrots, beetroot, turnip, parsnips, sweet potatoes, radishes and jerusalem artichokes.

FRUITS: Unlike vegetables, fruit has to be limited. Although nutritionally dense and good for you, it is sugar none the less and some fruits can be frighteningly high in this.

The best options are a mix of berries - strawberries, blueberries, blackberries, raspberries and cranberries, along with rhubarb and kiwi fruits. (Avocados and olives are also classed as fruits and are an excellent source of quality fats.)

NUTS: A must to add to your diet. Full of fibre, good fats and protein, they are the the perfect snack. Again the variety is there, so make the most of it. Experiment and keep it fresh. Try almonds, walnuts, pecans, pistachios, cashews, brazil nuts and hazelnuts for example.

FATS: Eggs, avocado, nuts, oily fish, olives, coconut and olive oils.

MEATS: Beef, chicken, turkey, pork, duck etc.

FISH : Tuna, salmon, sardines, trout, prawns, cod, mackerel, mussels, scallops

˙CONSUME IN LIMITED QUANTITIES

DAIRY: Milk, cheese, yoghurt (greek preferably, not low fat options)

FRUITS: High sugar fruits such as bananas, pineapples and mangoes along with fruit juices.

NON-WHEAT: Quinoa and oats.

PULSES: Beans (kidney, broad, black, butter), lentils and chickpeas.

CONSUME VERY RARELY OR PREFERABLY NEVER

Bread, pasta, noodles, cakes and biscuits, breakfast cereals, waffles, potatoes and rice

Dried fruits such as dates, prunes and raisins.

Sugary snacks such as sweets, energy bars, cereal bars and icecream.

Condiments such as jellies, jams, ketchups and shop-bought sauces.

Alcohol

FOOD AS MEDICINE

We see eating as something we need to do, to help us function and to give us energy to get through our busy days. This is true to a certain degree obviously. However, the food we eat has much more of an influence on our bodies than just controlling our body shape. It has a huge bearing on our health and is the cause and remedy of many of the illnesses, ailments, aches and pains we suffer from.

A simple way of terming it that I was taught was:

Your body is like a car. Put the wrong fuel in and it won't go far.

Some of the effects of eating foods that are wrong for our bodies are:

Nausea, vomiting, constipation, diarrhoea, stomach cramps, bloating, heartburn, gas, tiredness, fatigue, lethargy, headaches, faintness, insomnia, dizziness, aches and pains in joints and muscles, stiffness and feelings of weakness.

All of these symptoms can be cleared up or dramatically reduced by looking at what we eat. This is why fad diets and slimming clubs are not the answer. Firstly, as we have discussed, we want to lose fat not just weight, but also we want to feel great inside as well as looking great on the outside. Both go hand in hand. The better you are on the inside, the better you will become on the outside. We spend fortunes on products to make our skin, hair and nails look better, when this is better done by what we put in our bodies not on them.

Therefore we need to take our diet, our way of eating and personalise it.

Working from the food list above will dramatically change your body shape and wellbeing as this is made up of foods high in the nutrition that our body needs. We are giving it what it wants. However, then you must take it to the next stage and personalise it for you. As discussed, no two people are the same. We all have differing needs and requirements for our bodies. Our bodies react to different foods in different ways and you need to understand your own body in order to achieve the ultimate shape and wellbeing transformation.

You must look at what you eat and work out how it affects you. Look and see how you feel 60-120 minutes after eating. See if you feel bright and energetic or sluggish and tired. Are you bloated? Are you suffering from constipation or headaches? Do you wake up in the morning with aches and pains in certain areas or even all over your body? This can all be related back to foods that you have eaten or are eating. This is where you must take it to the next level and personalise your diet.

My own story of doing this came from a few symptoms where I was experiencing bloating along with aches and pains. So I did a week's food diary and marked down how I was feeling shortly after each meal I had. From it I saw a pattern of feeling sluggish after porridge (oats and milk) and red meat. After doing some research on these items I discovered that milk and oats can cause these symptoms as it is suggested that both are not natural to our bodies and therefore can cause digestive issues which could be what I was suffering from. Red meat is also hard for your stomach to break down and some people do suffer as a result of this.

On the other hand, I found that after eating scrambled eggs for breakfast instead of porridge and on days where I had fish instead of meat, I felt much better, these symptoms were not evident and my energy levels stayed more consistent throughout the day. The answer was simple : eradicate these items from my diet and eradicate the issues.

A common response from clients is that these are foods they enjoy. This is understandable and I agree it is not easy to give up foods that we enjoy, but it was about looking at the bigger picture for myself and asking whether it was worth the uncomfortable pains I was experiencing just to have a steak sandwich or a glass of milk.

As I said before, the best person to listen to for enabling you to eat the proper diet is you, your own body. It will tell you exactly what you need to give it for it to function at its optimum level, to change in shape and to maintain the changes.

Next we will look at two of the most common foods that people find they are allergic to to some degree ; dairy and wheat.

WHEAT

Most people have become (or are becoming) aware that white bread is not good for us and they steer more towards brown when making their purchase. Evidence shows however that brown bread is just as bad.

As mentioned above, according to the glycaemic index, which compares the effects of carbohydrates on our blood sugar levels, bread, both white and brown, is *higher than normal table sugar*.

Diets high in wheat from foods such as bread, wraps, cakes, cookies, pastries, pasta, pizza, breaded and battered foods, cereals, canned soups and beer have been shown to contribute to illnesses such as obesity, digestive diseases and arthritis.

My own experience of removing wheat from my diet had extraordinary effects on my health. The first thing to improve was that my bloating greatly reduced. This was something that had troubled me for many years, for as long as I could remember. By the end of some days I could hardly button my jeans up and was in continuous pain from it, but at the time I never made the link. Why would I ? Bread is constantly promoted as healthy, wholesome and nutritious. Immediately, I felt a big difference just from cutting back on them, but still I had toast with my breakfast and sandwiches when I was in a hurry. Still these problems were there, not as prevalent, but still niggling away.

When I finally took the plunge and totally removed bread from my diet I was amazed by the results. Within three weeks the changes were huge. The aches, pains and stiffness that I felt each morning upon wakening where gone. I had put these down to getting older or not enough stretching after my training each day. However, I was wrong. It had been down to the food I was eating. These issues were gone, my stomach was flatter than ever and the cramps I often experienced were also gone.

How can this supposedly healthy food that we are told to make the cornerstone of our diet actually be causing us so many issues?   Because the whole wheat that we eat today has been greatly modified from the natural grain it begins life as. The changes being made to our modern grains have now made it something that our bodies are just not designed to be able to digest properly, especially in the amounts we are eating.

Coeliac disease is an intense sensitivity to wheat that we all know about, which causes severe cramping and diahorrea, but even those who do not suffer to this extent may still be experiencing a level of intolerance to it.

The constant rise and fall of blood sugar levels from eating a high wheat diet stimulates the appetite meaning we are constantly craving and feeling hungry, meaning we are often overeating and normally it's the wrong things we are overindulging in and this is what creates health problems.

The best way to break the habit is to gradually decrease your intake. Start by changing your breakfast, eradicating it from that meal, lunches next and so on. You will experience cravings for it, which is normal, however the benefits far outweigh this.

As I say, after cutting it from my diet, the changes I felt were quite unbelievable. However the interesting part is now I cannot actually eat wheat, as within 45-90 minutes I will be doubled over in pain with stomach cramps, which just goes to show how much damage it had been doing to my body for all the years I was eating it 3-4 times a day.

Listen to your body and you will not go far wrong.

DAIRY

With regards to milk and dairy products, the first question is: Why do we eat and drink them? This is an example of one of those occasions where we need to question information and not just follow it blindly. Ask yourself why we are drinking milk from cows and goats.

Cows' milk is for young cows, goats' milk is for young goats, and human milk is for our babies. Why did we begin to drink milk meant for other animals? Why is it acceptable to drink milk from certain animals such as cows and goats, but not from other animals?

Milk is something I have removed from my diet. Noticing I felt sluggish mid-morning on certain days, I looked at what I was eating for breakfast on these days, saw it was porridge and tried taking milk and oats out of my diet for a while to gauge the results. I felt a lot better and my sluggishness went. I had always had a touch of eczema which I had used a cream for, prescribed by my doctor. After withdrawing milk from my diet, the eczema disappeared and I was able to stop using the medication that I had been on for years.

On one occasion with someone I was working with I asked if they would take milk from a breastfeeding woman and use that in their tea or coffee and I was met by a horrified expression. Why then do you take milk from an animal but not from a natural source to humans?

Now, I am not saying you should not drink milk ever again or that you are intolerant to it, but what I am saying and what I say to all my clients is this: question what you eat and drink. Look at things closely and see how it affects you. Maybe it does you harm or perhaps it doesn't, but you need to look at everything and find this out for yourself. Symptoms of this could be bloating, diahorrea or stomach cramps. Do you suffer from any of these? If so, look at what you are eating and drinking and eradicate what the cause is.

Question everything and personalise your diet for you and your body, as no two people are exactly the same.

TREAT YOURSELF

When we look at changing our eating habits to make physical changes to our bodies, we go from one extreme to the next.

One day we think 'That's it, I'm going on a diet' and we throw all (what we deem to be) the bad stuff out.

We are not going to touch chocolate/wine/takeaway (insert your foods of choice here) for one, two or three months. Our determination is admirable but it is ultimately deemed to failure.

It is okay to have chocolate. It is okay to have wine. It is okay to have takeaways.

The first question I always ask my clients regarding their eating is : Do You Want To Be Perfect? I've never had an answer of yes. My clients, and most people in general, do not want six packs. They do not want the perfect body. They want to lose some fat, have more energy and feel better about themselves. So if you do not want to be perfect you do not need to eat perfectly.

You will have your non-negotiables, the foods you love and do not want to give up. Mine were and are as discussed, chocolate and ice cream. I never go a day without eating chocolate. Why should I ? I love it and food is to be enjoyed! Have your bits of chocolate, have your glass of wine and have a takeaway and don't beat yourself up about it. If you want a six pack then yes these things will need to go, but if you are looking to make the changes mentioned above then you have the room to enjoy these items in moderation. Have chocolate, but not a full box. Have a glass of wine, but do not feel it necessary to finish the bottle. Enjoy a takeaway, but not every night. It's all about striking that balance.

And when you do fall off course and have a bad day, as we all do, you just get back on track the next day. Many times I have been tired/bored/fed up/stressed and demolished a big tub of ice cream or a box of chocolates. Was it bad for me? Of course, far too much sugar. But did I beat myself up for it? No, never. These things happen and will happen again. It's not the end of the world. I just got back to normal the next day and got back on course, trained and ate properly and I forgot about it.

Food is to be enjoyed so don't punish yourself over it. You will 'fail' many times - that is a guarantee. You would not be human if you didn't. But learn from it and move on and you will get to where you want to be.

CHAPTER 6

TRAINING

MAKE FITNESS AND ACTIVITY PART OF YOUR EVERYDAY LIFE

Make exercise just another part of your life. In order to get the best results do not treat it like a chore.

Firstly, we did not get out of shape in the space of a few weeks (for myself it was over many years) so we are not going to be back in perfect shape in just a few days or a couple of weeks. It will take time. There are no quick fixes and no seven day diets that shift a stone of fat. These are all fads and any weight lost is predominantly water.

It takes hard work, there is no point in lying about that, but the pay off is massive if you do it correctly and eventually this will become just another part of your daily and weekly routine.

Therefore to make exercise a part of everyday life, we must ditch the all or nothing attitude. We do not need to be slogging away for an hour to 90 minutes every day to get results. This will last a few weeks and then the novelty will wear off. A little exercise each day or a few times per week will make a huge difference in the long term both physically and for your wellbeing.

Do not let excuses get in the way. We are all busy, but should not be too busy to look after our health. Regular excuses are:

Too busy: Even the busiest of us can find 15-20 minutes in a day to do some kind of physical exercise.

Too tired: Exercise reduces fatigue and boosts energy levels in the long run and it will help you sleep better which will in turn make you feel more refreshed each morning and alert.

I am too old/I am too unfit: It is never too late to start. No matter your age or level of physical fitness there is always something you could be doing to improve your current condition.

LONG, SLOW CARDIO IS NOT THE ANSWER

When most people think about burning fat they turn to long, slow cardio, i.e. treadmills and stationary bikes (and elliptical trainers. Yes, a machine to replicate walking. Indoors!)

This is the biggest, most common misconception in getting fit and getting the body you want and will seriously hinder your progress. I have yet to meet a person who enjoys using these machines and they are one of the biggest wastes of time you can spend fitness wise.

If you decide that you want to use these machines and you think they will get you the body you want then ask yourself what kind of bodies that long, slow cardio athletes such as distance runners and cyclists have. Google them and see pictures. Is this how you want to look? If it is, then this may not be the book for you. Long, slow cardio will indeed burn fat but also muscle, giving you that skeletal look where your clothes just hang on you.

Firstly, as I said, I have yet to meet anyone who enjoys this type of exercise. If we do not enjoy something we do, in any walk of life, we will not do it to our highest capabilities. That is just human nature. So right away we are off to a bad start. Secondly, we do not use them correctly. Most people do not change the pre-programmed settings, so it is like running/walking/cycling/rowing on flat, easy ground (or water) which is not realistic as when we do these things outdoors there are different levels of ascent and descent involved. Also, the treadmill is helping you because the band going round is pulling your feet back as you run, meaning you use less energy to go the same distance i.e. if it says you have run 10km it is more likely you have run the equivalent of 5 or 6km.

To transform your body shape and fitness levels you need to transform your training methods. Doing the same thing over and over will give you the same results as you have now. To be different you need to train differently.

DO HIGH INTENSITY INTERVAL TRAINING (HIIT)

The main concept of HIIT is to train the body at different levels of intensity and not let it get used to training at the same level continuously. Long endurance activities like marathon running can cause muscle catabolism (the breakdown of muscle tissue). HIIT training does the opposite : it helps increase speed, power, endurance and metabolic rate, helping you burn fat faster.

As well as this, it is time efficient. Clients see amazing results in body shape and fitness levels with just 30 minutes of training. It is a way to get in, train and get out again in the minimum time necessary, but still get results, which is ideal as few people want, and need to be, in the gym for 60-90 minutes at a time.

It is also challenging both to the body and to the brain. One of the main reasons for failure in the gym is boredom. Running, cycling or rowing at the same pace for the same amount of time (some people even using the exact same piece of equipment each time - they have their 'own' machine) can become boring and monotonous, not just for our bodies but for our brains. Once this happens, our levels of application drop as it is hard to give 100% when we are bored and not stimulated.

My sessions of HIIT and HIIT in general keep your body guessing as well as your brain, training all different muscles from different angles and with different stimuli.

Try it the next time you visit the gym : change the speed and intensity at which you work. Work in intervals of 15 seconds at high intensity and 15-25 in recovery mode, then build this up so the rest time comes down as your fitness improves.

BUILD MUSCLE, USE WEIGHTS

By training with weights you will add muscle to your frame. The body has to burn more energy to carry muscle and it keeps your metabolic rate high, hence why you see athletes with greater muscle mass eating a greater quantity of food and not getting fat.

As we get older, from 30 years of age onwards, our bodies change and one of the biggest changes is that we begin to lose muscle. Everyone does. On average a person will lose between 5-8% of their muscle mass each decade from their 30s onwards. To counter this we must train with weights or some kind of resistance to maintain our muscle levels and if possible improve them.

When we put on excess weight, we panic and go for the treadmill. We run and run, thinking that this is the answer. This type of cardio burns *weight* in three forms: fat, muscle and water.

This means we are losing muscle from ageing and now from exercise. This, along with our diets low in protein from meat, chicken, fish, eggs, nuts etc. which are essential for muscle repair and growth, means we are losing muscle from three different angles. This muscle is being replaced on our bodies by fat.

Building muscle is imperative for you to have the body you want.

My type of training is not going to give you huge, hulking muscles, something that many women fear even though their bodies are not built to easily increase muscle mass. It will give you a lean, toned, athletic look, which is what most of us want.

WHY COMMERCIAL GYMS DO NOT WORK

As mentioned in *My Transformation Story,* gyms are not set up to get people results.

By their very nature, gyms should be full of healthy, fit people successfully improving themselves on each visit. In my time training in them, the majority of people using them did not fall into this category and now working in the industry, it is still the same.

Gyms are set up to make money, pure and simple. I am not saying there is anything wrong with this, it is a business after all and we are all looking to make money, but it is coming at the expense of client success, not hand in hand with it as it should. In my experience of these gyms, there are many issues that contribute to your lack of results.

The first one is the equipment. Now, we know that people are apprehensive and reluctant to both join and use gyms. This is understandable. Who would not be slightly scared of doing something they do not know much about? So in order to make these gyms attractive and less intimidating they get filled with nice, safe, easy looking machines. Running machines (we know how to run or walk) and bikes (yes, we know how to cycle). We see this as safe, we have used similar equipment before, we will not make a fool of ourselves and we head straight for them.

The majority of the rest of the gym is full of weight machines. These are machines where you sit and carry out isolation moves on your legs, arms, back, chest etc. Again they look safe and cosy and we get a seat so as not to stand out as we want to be inconspicuous. They don't want you to feel awkward as you may cancel your membership. The area where the majority of gains will be made is in the smallest part of the gym, the free weights section. Rarely will anyone in a gym wander into this section without assistance as it is intimidating and normally full of big blokes and big weights. So we stick to the 95% of the gym that looks comfortable and where we will not look out of place.

However, ask your trainer or anyone working in the gym how often they use these machines and if they are truthful they will tell you never. They are actively encouraging you to use items of equipment that are not good enough for them to train with but they seem to think it is good enough for you, the paying client.

The second issue is the price and the amount of members. I have seen big gyms, with plenty of machines, however when full to capacity, they will hold no more than 500-600 people. However they have between 5000 and 6000 members. So they have set up a gym that cannot hold all its members should they all come along. However, they know that all their members will never come along. They know there will never be a need for 500+ people to be catered for because they set up their business to ensure that the majority of people rarely set foot in the gym.

They keep the price so low that thousands join, because it makes people believe they are taking steps to get fit. They keep the price so low that you will not cancel. It's only 10/12/15 pounds per month, too much hassle to cancel, I'll just leave it as I will definitely go back next month when I am not so busy with (insert reason here). So they know that of 6000 members maybe 1000 will be regular users, and by making it open 24 hours, they know it is unlikely (they have done research) that all 1000 will come at the same time.

So they receive the £10/12/15 from each member each month and do not care if they never see them again, as they know the cancellation rate is so small, so the income stays big.

The third reason for failure is the people being employed there. This is no slight on the trainers there, many are very good at what they do, but the environment is not set up for their success either.

For one thing, they do not get paid by the gym they work in. *They are freelance, working for themselves within that gym.* They do 12-15 hours of work for the gym, doing inductions, cleaning and generally being on hand in exchange for not having to pay rental costs to use the gym facility in order to train their own clients. Basically unless you are paying them for personal training, they have little interest in what you are doing in the gym. They have no incentive to come and advise you (understandably, who wants to work for free), to help you with mistakes you are making or improvements you could make to your training (unless they think they can convert you to becoming a paying client). To sum up, this is an excellent business model, but a shameful fitness model. To transform your body you may need to think laterally.

THINK DIFFERENTLY

If you do not enjoy going to the gym, why do you do it??

I made this mistake for many months and years before I decided to go and explore other avenues and find what I enjoy doing and it is essential that you do this too. As is human nature, when you do something you love, you will do it better, be more committed to it and get improved results by it.

Question why you use the gym. Do you enjoy it? Could you be doing something different and more beneficial? What would you do fitness wise if you had a choice of anything at all? Ask yourself these questions and they will help you find the best way to get fit for you personally.

For me, it was my love of sports and admiration for these athletes. How did they do it? What was the secret? Could I imitate them? Here, I will give you some information on the techniques I use for myself and for my clients to get maximum success:

Battleropes: A brutally effective way of burning fat and conditioning your body, replacing the antiquated idea of the need to do long distance running or steady state cardio as the best way to do this. It is also low impact, meaning less stress on your joints. Ropes will not only build muscles in your shoulders, arms and core, but you'll simultaneously burn fat around these muscles as well.

Kettlebells: Kettlebell training has many benefits. Along with the extremely high metabolic cost of throwing the weight around, this type of training also creates dense muscle mass. There is no better way to burn fat than with a few sets of kettlebell swings, snatches and clean & jerks. They will give you an all-in-one workout of a lifetime, combining both strength and cardio aspects.

Sandbag training: Sandbags share a lot in common   with kettlebells in regards to their ability to challenge not only strength, but endurance as well. The bag allows for movement of the sand within, therefore forcing the lifter to manoeuvre and adjust to the awkward weight. This definitely causes the body to use more muscles and expend greater energy as it is hard to get into one consistent groove.

TRX suspension training : This engages the whole body. The instability that the straps create whilst you perform movements means that your core is constantly activated. Moreover, the functional movements mean that many muscles are worked   at the same time, providing a very comprehensive, all-over workout.

Medicine balls : These are a great way to exercise any area of your body, whether upper, lower, or core. There are many advantages to training with medicine balls. They allow for improved range of motion, core strength, coordination, flexibility, joint integrity and upper and lower body strength.

These are what I found I enjoyed and my results rocketed immediately once I started using them. Maybe they will be for you, maybe they will not, but it is essential that you find what you enjoy doing in order to get the maximum results possible and reach your goals.

WORK YOUR BODY AS ONE

As discussed, in the majority of gyms you will find that the space is taken up by treadmills, stationary bikes, rowing machines and weight machines to work legs, arms, shoulders etc. in isolation.

From gym owners and employees, you are encouraged as gym members to use this equipment with the promise that they will get you results. However to get (and maintain) lean muscle and keep body fat low, you need to be doing full body moves.

These include deadlifts, squats, cleans, snatches, lunges, split squats etc.

Working major muscles together in compound moves such as these requires more energy and works more of the major muscles which gets bigger results quicker. By choosing compound exercises to make up the majority of your routine, you will ensure you are getting the most intense workout

possible. This also means less time in the gym and who wants to be training any more than is necessary for maximum results?

We are all busy and have other commitments to take care of so making your sessions up of multiple muscle exercises will cut the time you need to spend training considerably.

INTENSITY

As discussed previously, only 20% of your results will come from what you do in the minutes and hours you spend in the gym. However this is not to say that training is not important. It is essential for you to get the results you want.

Over time I have observed people 'training' incorrectly. I did it myself for many years, so I know the signs. We spend an hour plus in the gym. However we actually train for about 15/20 minutes. The rest of the time is spent: texting, checking facebook, watching television, chatting, wandering about, looking at what other people are doing. Basically wasting time. With the 15/20 minutes we do actually train, we do so at a level so low it has minimum effect on our bodies.

As we now know, we break our bodies down in the gym. However this only happens with the correct intensity, which few of us use. To put it simply our muscles are made up of many small fibres. When we train at the correct intensity we tear these fibres. At this point we have succeeded in our goal of going to the gym and the work outside the gym now kicks in.

If we do not work at the proper intensity then we do not break the muscles. At best we stretch/strain them a bit, but we do not tear them. Therefore even if we eat correctly, we will not see the physical changes that we desire as the intensity was not there to break the body down in order for the food and rest to take over and build our muscles back up bigger and stronger.

So when you go to the gym leave all phones and distractions at home or in your locker and only train with someone who has the same goals as you, because as much fun as it is to be there with a friend, if they are keeping you from training to achieve your best results then it is not going to work.

WHY YOU MUST STRIVE TO FAIL

Just as we attempt to break muscle, not build muscle in the gym, we also must strive to fail in the gym before we will see success. This is something many clients find strange, but let me explain.

As discussed, where most people fail in their fitness and body change goals is doing the wrong exercise for what they want and not working with the proper intensity. The third part of the issue is they do not push themselves to fail. This part is important because even with the other two parts in place you must fail in the gym to get results.

I see people train within the gym environment and can tell just by looking at them that they are coasting along and working well within themselves. People are of the mindset that if it is easier (or becoming easier) then they are getting fitter. This is a major mistake. I have had clients whom when telling me about a fitness class they have attended have been embarrassed as they are puffing and exhausted by the end and yet they see other people walk by who look as though they have hardly broken sweat. They aspire to be like these people because "Well, they must be very fit then surely?". However these people won't be getting any fitter, they will remain where they are until they push themselves on beyond these boundaries, but they don't want to as they are 'afraid to fail'.

The example I give to clients to hit this point home is:

If they were to train with me, the two of us together, then I could probably work at around 70-80% of my capacity to my client's 100% and still be faster, get more reps in, lift heavier weights and to someone watching I would be the 'better' of the two training. However, only one of us would be improving. My client would be getting better as they are working to their maximum, they are pushing themselves to failure, getting every last lift, push, pull, lunge and squat into their session. This would get them results and they would see themselves improving each session. A few sessions later they would be getting one more rep in, lifting a little bit more weight, feeling stronger for longer instead of feeling spent midway through the session. Whereas I would still be lifting the same weights and getting in the same reps in the work time. Basically I would be where I was weeks earlier, at best maintaining my fitness.

Yes, I would look fresher at the end of the session than my client would, but only because I would have been coasting throughout the session, working well within myself, not pushing myself beyond my limits ; playing it safe. Only one of us would be transforming our body, seeing our fitness levels improve, building more muscle and heading towards our goals.

Another thing clients always comment to me about is "Why is this not getting any easier ? Am I not getting fitter?". It should never get easier. It will never get easier. You should always be looking to fail. Once you can lift 10kg comfortably then you need to push to 11kg. You may not get as many reps in at 11kg, but you keep practicing and one day you will. You keep failing until the day comes when you do lift it 8 times for example, then you push the weight up again to a weight where you fail at 7 reps and you keep trying, keep failing. Once you can manage 6 lunges in the work time, you should strive to make 7. Two of us working together at our maximum will have us both exhausted at the end of the training session equally because we have both given 100%, whatever our respective 100% is. If we do this, we will both be improving.

So it is imperative that you do not coast through a session. Doing the same thing will only get you the same results. Making sure you fail is a sure step to success.

ONE ON ITS OWN WILL NOT DO

To build and maintain the body, health and wellbeing we want, we need the full 100% of eating and training together. One without the other just will not work.

Eat well without training and you will cut fat, but you will not get the shape you want as you won't build the muscle you desire to give you shape and definition.

Train without eating properly and you will get fitter, your cardiovascular levels will improve and you will improve your muscle mass and strength but it will be buried under a layer of fat and you will not be able to see the gains you have made.

Both of these areas work hand in hand and both together are needed for ultimate success. Your body was designed to eat and process certain foods and to prosper from them. It was designed to move as a whole and on a regular basis.

Give your body what it wants and needs and it will repay you.

CHAPTER SEVEN

AND FINALLY......

Although I have said success comes from 80% food and 20% training, there are a couple of other factors that are vitally important in your transformation and these are sleep and hydration.

SLEEP

As we now know, our transformation success will come from eating the correct food to repair the torn muscles that our correct training has given us. However the main time when this healing (and growth) of the muscles will take place is when we sleep.

The importance of sleep is vitally important to your success in a couple of ways:

Growth: When we are sleeping our body is recovering from the wear and tear inflicted on it from our daily activities. If we have provided it with the proper foods, our body will repair itself and muscles will grow while we are at rest. This is why the myth of not eating after 6/7pm is nonsense.

Let's say you last ate at 7pm and your next meal is breakfast at 7am. That is a 12 hour gap between foods. Would you go 12 hours during the day without eating? If you had breakfast at 7am, could you happily not eat again until 7pm? Would you be able to function at your work and during training with no food for 12 hours?? Well, your body is still working while you sleep and needs sustenance to do so.

Therefore it is important to have some protein based food not long before you go to sleep. Nothing heavy that is going to   sit uncomfortably as you try to sleep, but something for your body to use to help it repair itself.

At the same time, the old saying that breakfast is the most important meal of the day is very true. Again, if you wake up and skip breakfast and do not eat until nearer lunch, your body would again have had, depending on when your last meal before bed was, far too long a gap between meals thus depriving it of the essential nutrients needed to sufficiently build it.

The second important reason to get adequate sleep is because we will function better as we will have more energy and our cravings will be less. The times when I am most tempted to break away from my way of eating are when I am tired. When I wake up after too short or a disturbed sleep and I am still tired, these are the days when I am more likely to grab for sugary snacks to give myself that boost to get me through my busy day.

Getting that proper rest gives you the energy to get up feeling properly refreshed and ready for the day ahead. It gives me the energy to train harder and to prepare my meals and therefore get better results. It is all one big circle with everything linked towards gaining success. Alternatively, not getting proper sleep leads to being tired and irritable, being less likely to handle the events of the day, reaching for sugary junk food for an 'energy boost' and then feeling bad at the inevitable sugar crash/energy dip and the fact that you have broken your good eating plans. This will make you less likely to train, and so the vicious circle continues.

HYDRATION

Our bodies are made up of 55-60% water. Our brain function and physical abilities can start to be affected by just a 1% drop in hydration. Effects can be headaches, loss of concentration, lethargy, dry skin, constipation and invariably overeating.

Staying hydrated is one of the most important ways to stay healthy and maintain the body shape you want. However, most of us are dehydrated without even realising it.

The key is to not wait until you feel thirsty before you drink water. Continuously sipping water throughout the day is the secret to ensuring proper hydration.

When we are dehydrated our bodies receive mixed signals. We feel tired and think we need to eat for more energy whereas what we really need is water. This leads to overeating (again, usually the wrong things) and so problems ensue.

However, sugar-filled juices, teas and coffees should not be used as a substitute for water. If you find water too bland, add some fresh fruit to it in a jug overnight to infuse the flavours and then drink it throughout the day. If you still enjoy tea or coffee then ensure you drink a glass of water along with it to counter the dehydration caused.

CONCLUSION

This is the knowledge and information I have used to transform my body shape, fitness levels and health to a level I have never seen before.

These are the techniques I have used to train many clients to amazing results and transformations in only 12 weeks and then to carry this on beyond into the months and years that follow. It works, and not only is it the best way to get the body you want, more importantly it is the best way to *maintain* the transformation well after the 12 weeks.

I would like to thank you for taking the time to read my book and hope it was informative and that you got something from it. I would love to hear your stories of how you got on with your transformation and would be delighted to answer   any questions on the matter.

Feel free to contact me through my website :

www.theguerrillacoach.co.uk

Good luck!

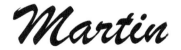

Martin

RECIPES
(A few ideas to get you started...)

SIMPLE SCRAMBLED EGGS

2-3 Eggs
Butter
Cream
Chives

- Crack the eggs into a cold pan and add a bit of butter. Transfer pan to the heat and begin to stir.

- Continue to stir, whilst moving the pan on and off the heat regularly to prevent eggs overheating and becoming rubbery.

- Take the eggs off the heat when they are still a little runny (as the residual heat of the pan will finish them off).

- Add a spoonful of cream (this will help prevent eggs overcooking) along with seasoning and chives and fold in.

- Add or serve with option of mushrooms, spinach, cherry tomatoes, grilled bacon bits, different cheeses etc. Experiment!

TOMATO AND CHORIZO SALAD

3 Large ripe tomatoes (cut into wedges) or 12 cherry
tomatoes (halved)
Half a red onion, sliced thinly
A few sprigs of fresh thyme
1 Tablespoon of sherry vinegar
2 Tablespoons of olive oil
100g Chorizo, sliced

- Put the tomatoes in a bowl with thyme. Season, then drizzle with the vinegar and the oil. Let the flavours infuse.

- Add the chorizo to a hot, dry pan and slowly begin to fry the chorizo slices.

- When some of the oil is released, add the onion and cook until chorizo is browned on both sides and onion has softened. Mix all together and serve the tomatoes with the fried chorizo, drizzled with a little oil from the pan.

MACKEREL PATE

300g Mackerel
150g Cream cheese
1 Lime, juice & zest
Fresh chives or dill
Sea salt & pepper

- Cut up the mackerel into small pieces and add to a large bowl.

- Add the cheese, juice & zest along with the herbs and season well.

- Using a large spoon, mix it all together.

- Transfer to an airtight container and keep in the fridge.

- Alternatives: A spoonful of horseradish, lemon or parsley.

- Serve with   carrot or celery sticks and/or sundried tomatoes.

BROCCOLI CHEESE SOUP

3 Broccoli heads
2 Onions, chopped roughly
2 Celery sticks, chopped
1 Leek, chopped
Chicken stock
Cheese of choice (for me, it's blue, but not everyone's cup of tea!)
Olive oil

- Peel and chop up the onions and add to pan when oil is sizzling. Cook for a few minutes until starting to soften.

- Add celery and leek, lightly season and stir and cook for a further few minutes.

- Add broccoli.

- Pour in enough stock to just cover. Bring to the boil and then simmer for 10-12 mins until broccoli has softened.

- Remove some of the stock. (Tip: Too much stock can make it too watery. Keep stock to one side and add more if too thick for your preference. Remember, you can always add ingredients while cooking but cannot take them away!)

- Blend with stick blender.

- Add cheese to taste, a little at a time. Blend and taste (see tip above!). Season to taste if needing more.

CARROT AND SWEET POTATO MASH

300g Sweet potato, peeled and cut into chunks
300g Carrots, washed and cut into chunks
2 Garlic cloves, chopped - add salt and crush into a paste
Cumin
Coriander
Sea salt & pepper
Knob of butter

- Cut vegetables to roughly same-sized pieces to ensure an even cook. Add to a pan, cover with water, bring to the boil and then simmer until soft but not mushy (between 10-15 minutes depending on how small you have cut the vegetables).

- Drain and add the garlic paste along with the cumin and/or coriander and season well.

- Mash everything up, add the butter and check for seasoning. Continue to mash until everything is combined. Serve immediately or place in a bowl and cover with clingfilm to reheat later.

COD WITH CREAMY LEEKS & BACON

2 x 150g Cod fillets skin on and seasoned with sea salt &
freshly ground black pepper
Olive oil or coconut oil
Large knob of butter
3 Rashers streaky bacon, cut into thin strips
1.5 Medium sized leeks cut into slices
60ml (5fl oz) Double cream
Parmesan cheese, grated
Salt & pepper to season

- Heat the olive or coconut oil in a large frying pan.
  Once it begins to sizzle, place the fish in skin side
  down. Leave to cook for a few minutes or until fish is
  cooked ¾ of the way through (you will see the colour
  change from bottom upwards). Turn it over and remove
  from the heat. The residual heat in the pan will continue
  to cook the fish.

- Heat a large saucepan and add some oil and once
  sizzling add the bacon. Fry for a few minutes until it's
  golden and crisp.

- Transfer the bacon to a plate and stir in the leeks. Cook
  for a few minutes or until tender. Take off the heat,
  pour over the cream and stir until lightly thickened (the
  heat of the pan will be enough).

- Stir through the parmesan and bacon. To serve, spoon
  the leeks onto a serving plate and top with the fish.

CHICKEN ONE TRAY BAKE

8 Chicken thighs
4 Garlic cloves, peeled and finely chopped
2 Red Peppers, deseeded and chopped
2 Green Peppers, deseeded and chopped
2 Yellow Peppers, deseeded and chopped
Jar of pitted black olives
4 Red onions, peeled and chopped into chunks
Mixture of thyme, parsley, basil and/or oregano
1 Tablespoon of paprika
200g Chorizo, cut into chunks
200g Cherry tomatoes
1 Tin of chopped tomatoes
Splash of sherry vinegar or red wine vinegar

- Add all ingredients except the chicken into a large bowl or pan and mix together. Season well with sea salt and pepper.

- Tip into baking tray and add the chicken pieces, skin side up, nestled into the vegetable mix.

- Place into an oven that has been preheated to 190°C and cook for 35 minutes or until chicken is cooked through. Check by putting knife into chicken. If cooked through, juice should run out clear.

Recommended Books:

The following are books that I have read, enjoyed, found extremely informative and that have helped form the basis of my knowledge and opinions on the matters above. If you wish to take your reading further and delve deeper into these subjects, I would recommend them.

Fat Chance by Dr Robert Lustig

Wheat Belly by Dr William Davis

Eat Fat Get Thin by Dr Mark Hyman

Why Am I Not Losing Weight by Pete Cohen

The 21 Day Sugar Detox by Diane Sanfilippo

Serve to Win by Novak Djokovic

Printed in Great Britain
by Amazon

82608556R00068